Turmeric: Improve Your Cooking, Health & Wellness with This Miracle Spice

By Francine Agile

Table of Contents

Copyright

The information provided herein is stated to be truthful and consistent, in that any liability, in terms of inattention or otherwise, by any usage or abuse of any policies, processes, or directions contained within is the solitary and utter responsibility of the recipient reader.

Under no circumstances will any legal responsibility or blame be held against the publisher for any reparation, damages, or monetary loss due to the information herein, either directly or indirectly.

Respective authors own all copyrights not held by the publisher.

The information herein is offered for informational purposes solely and is universal as so. The presentation of the information is without contract or any type of guarantee assurance.

The trademarks that are used are without any consent, and the publication of the trademark is without permission or backing by the trademark owner. All trademarks and brands within this book are for clarifying purposes only and are the owned by the owners themselves, not affiliated with this document.

Introduction

This book contains lots of information about turmeric, the spice that's been widely popular today because of its taste and health benefits.

Have you ever wondered where curry dishes get that yellowish hue? Yes, that's from turmeric. People widely recognize turmeric in curry, however, they seldom know that turmeric has many other uses and can be present in other dishes and things. There's actually a lot more to this spice than making a curry dish tasty and colorful.

The goal of this book is to provide you with more information about turmeric. Here, you will learn this spice's history, cooking uses, and amazing benefits to your health and well-being.
Once you've known how turmeric works for your health, feel free to include turmeric in your daily dishes! There's a special chapter dedicated to easy-to-prepare delicious turmeric recipes so that you can experience the goodness of turmeric in your daily meals.

So, are you now ready to discover what else turmeric can do aside from tickling your taste buds? Go ahead and read on! Turmeric isn't dubbed *"Miracle Spice"* for nothing!

Thanks for purchasing this book, I hope you enjoy it!

Chapter 1: What is Turmeric?

Let us start to familiarize ourselves with turmeric by learning about its definition, physical appearance, and other attributes. We will also learn about its common uses and how the plant is cultivated.

Definition of Turmeric

Turmeric is an herbaceous root that comes from a plant called *Curcuma longa*. Turmeric is a close cousin of ginger, and they both belong in the same ginger family known botanically as *Zingiberaceae*.

Turmeric is a rhizome, which means each tubular root has the ability to grow into another set of turmeric plants when re-planted onto the soil. Plant shoots grow again from the bud protrusions on the turmeric roots.

Etymology of Turmeric

It is uncertain where the name turmeric truly came from. Popular belief dictates that the term came from two different Middle English words *turmeryte* or *tarmaret*, and the Medieval Latin words *terra merita* which all mean *"merited earth"*.

Physical Appearance

Turmeric plants have erect olive green-colored leaves that shoot upwards from fat and thick stems. The leaves are tapered down to its ends. Turmeric plants can grow more than three feet tall, depending on the soil conditions or the plant itself. Turmeric flowers may vary from yellow, white, and pink in color and blossom around a month after planting the rhizomes.

The rhizome roots share a strikingly similar appearance with their close cousin ginger. A typical turmeric root is generally brownish, tubular, and oval in shape. It also has bud protrusions around it. Each root is typically 2 to 3 inches long and almost an inch thick. Turmeric has a fleshy yet hard interior that is brownish-orange in color. Some varieties may even have rust-colored interior flesh.

Turmeric roots are dense and can easily be broken down into fine lemon-gold colored powder when they are completely dried.

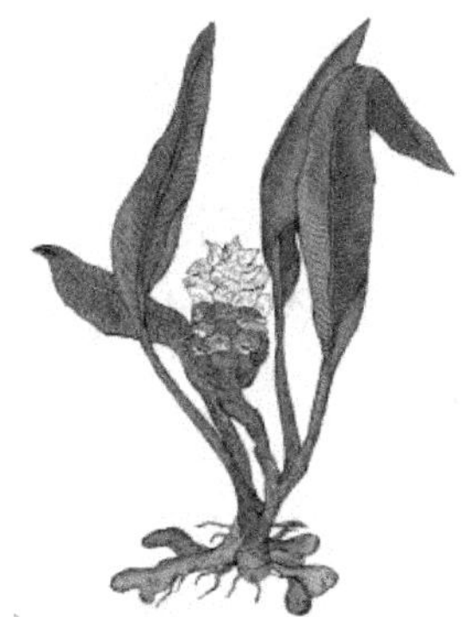
An Illustration of a Turmeric Plant

Nutrient Content

Turmeric roots contain the following vitamins, minerals, and compounds:

- Copper

- Manganese

- Iron

- Fiber

- Potassium

- Phosphorus8

- Vitamin B6

- Calcium chloride

- Starches

- Curcumin

Curcumin stands out the most among all these nutrient contents. Curcumin is a compound that gives turmeric its bright golden-yellow color. It is also seen as the most nutritious substance in turmeric, giving the rhizome properties that make it beneficial for human health.

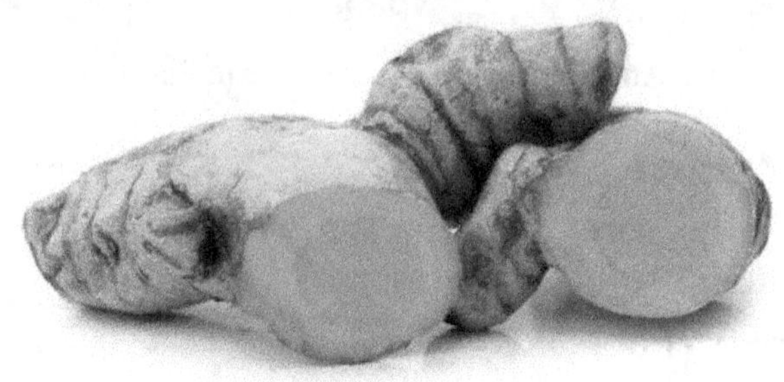

Turmeric's Flavor

Contrary to popular belief, turmeric isn't a spicy herb. Perhaps that belief came from the fact that the herb is often used to make spicy curry dishes. In reality, turmeric has a slightly bitter and pepper-like flavor. It also has a strong biting taste closely similar to ginger. Fresh turmeric has a slightly sweet and nutty taste and a chewy texture that masks the bitterness and makes it more palatable. Turmeric warms the mouth and stains the saliva, tongue, and teeth with a golden yellow tint when eaten.

Cultivating Turmeric Plants

Turmeric plants can be grown indoors on pots before transferring them in an outside garden or planting area.

Turmeric rhizome roots are gathered and planted on warm, well-drained, neutral soil. Each rhizome should ideally contain plenty of buds (those bumps alongside the turmeric's sides) to produce more plants. Rhizomes can be cut so that each one has two to three buds in it before being planted in the soil.

Turmeric likes warmth and sunshine and thrives in temperatures ranging from 68 to 86 degrees Fahrenheit. Plant turmeric in a colder environment, and the rhizomes would likely rot instead of sprout. Despite this intolerance for cold temperatures, the plant can tolerate annual rainfall in most tropical areas like in India, Indonesia, Taiwan, China, Bangladesh, Sri Lanka, and the Philippines.

Plant sprouts will begin to appear within a week. Continue caring for the turmeric plants until they are ready for harvest, usually 7 to 10 months from the initial planting period. You'll know harvest time has come when the stems and leaves start to appear brownish and dried.

Common Uses of Turmeric

Turmeric is widely known in the culinary world as an herbal spice in powder form used to season curries and other succulent dishes. The spice is extensively used as a condiment in Indian, East Asian, and Southeast Asian cuisine.

Apart from its culinary significance, turmeric has many more uses such as:
- an alternative to toxic food and medicine colorings

- a substitute for saffron in some dishes

- a preservative that prolongs the shelf life of foods and oils such as sesame oil and olive oil

- a fabric dye in many Indian regions

- an important ingredient in manufacturing papers used to test for the alkalinity of solutions

- a key ingredient in skin lotions and creams

- a cure in Eastern and Oriental medicine

Turmeric roots can be used fresh and can also be turned into powder. Several commercial preparations of turmeric are also available nowadays.

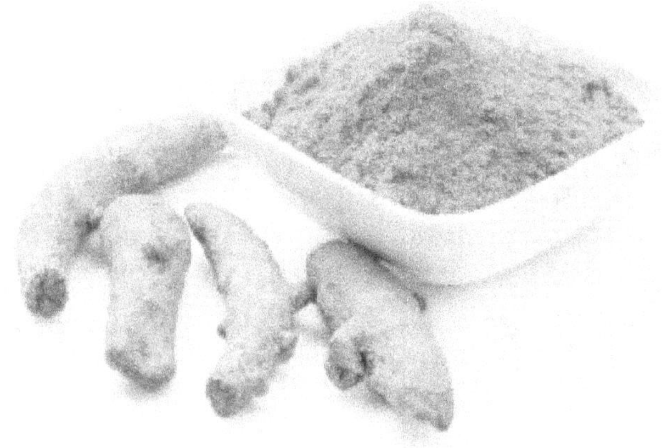

Chapter 2: The History of Turmeric

The humble turmeric plant has a rich history and is utilized extensively in the early days for a variety of uses. Eastern parts of the globe have known turmeric since the very beginning of time. However, Western discovery of turmeric did not begin until the dawn of the modern era. This explains why turmeric is becoming popular in the Western world only recently.

Where it all Began

Turmeric plants originated mainly from Southern India and Indonesia. The plant has been extensively cultivated and used by native Indians as part of Ayurveda, the ancient Indian medicinal science.
Ayurvedic medicine used turmeric for relieving arthritis, cough, flatulence, and indigestion. Ancient Indians also found that consuming turmeric root improves blood circulation, keeps the heart healthy, and increases energy. Turmeric's medicinal uses were documented in an Ayurveda compendium text published in 250 BC. Sanskrit texts in the 5th and 6th centuries AD also feature the various uses of turmeric.

Indians believed that the plant was a gift from the gods, and thus considered turmeric as a "divine" plant. Hence, turmeric held a special role in most Vedic rituals. The plant is extensively used in fertility ceremonies, weddings, and rituals for well-being.

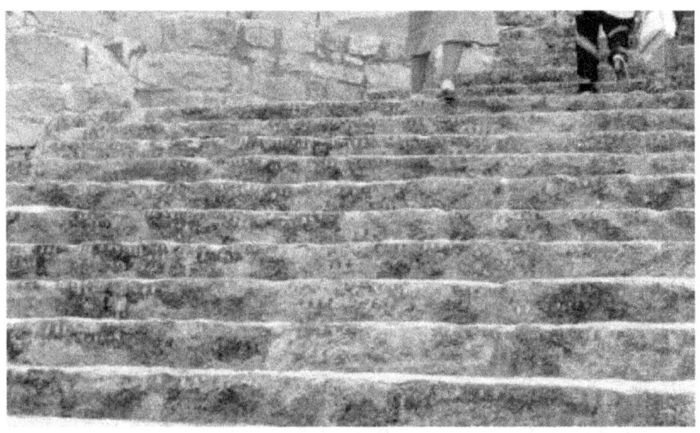

Decorated Indian Hindu steps with turmeric and kumkum

The following rituals involved the use of turmeric as part of worship:
- Haldi ceremony / Gaye holud, a festive ritual during wedding ceremonies of Hindus and Muslims in South Asia
- Kankanabandhana, a wedding ceremony in western India where turmeric tubers are tied to the couple's wrists

- Tamil-Telugu marriage rituals, where turmeric tubers are used in creating Thali necklaces (a representation of wedding bands in ancient Indian culture)
- Navapatrika worship during Durga festival rituals

Turmeric Cultivation and Use

Cultivation and spread of turmeric is significantly slower than those of seeded plants because turmeric rhizomes need to depend on the movement of people in order to be planted and spread on to other areas.

Babylon and Egypt

The plant is believed to be cultivated in the Gardens of Babylon in the early 8th century BC.   In 1500 BC, Egyptians started to use turmeric plants to heal wounds and dye skin and fabrics. Egyptian turmeric use is documented in the Ebers Papyrus, one of the world's earliest known records of using plants for medicinal purposes.

China

Turmeric spread to China during the Tang Dynasty (618-907 AD) and is locally known as jiang huang plant. Turmeric is used in traditional Chinese medicine to reduce inflammation, treat traumatic wound injuries, relieve abdominal pain, and help cure menstrual irregularities in women. The Chinese also believed that turmeric helps move the Qi and the blood properly.

Turmeric was included in China's Tang Materia Medica, the first published pharmacopoeia in the world. The book was compiled during the Tang Dynasty in 659 AD.

Buddhist monks also used turmeric to give their robes a bright yellowish-orange hue. As these monks travel constantly across Asia, they were also credited as propagators of turmeric use in nearby Asian countries.

Hawaii and other Tropical Countries

Hawaiians used turmeric to treat various illnesses, such as stomach ulcers, ear infections, nasal congestion, and sinus infections.

Other tropical countries in the Southeast part of Asia also started cultivating turmeric and used it as a dye and a medicinal plant. Turmeric is also included in several dishes in Indonesia, Cambodia, and Vietnam.

Africa

Turmeric reached East Africa in the early 800 AD, spread to West Africa by 1200 AD, then finally reached Jamaica in the 18th century. From there, turmeric use across the entire continent flourished continuously. Africans used turmeric for a variety of purposes:

- Dye for fabrics and clothes
- Food coloring for cheeses, margarine, butter, and yogurts
- Preparation of dishes such as geelrys (yellow rice)

The warm climate in most African countries contributed to the steady cultivation of turmeric plants in the entire region. Nowadays, African countries such as Kenya, Jamaica, Haiti, Nigeria, and South Africa grow and export turmeric products.

Middle East

When turmeric use flourished in India in the ancient times, neighboring Arabic countries also began to cultivate the plant. They used turmeric just a few years after the Indians started doing so.
Arabs are the ones who introduced turmeric use in the European continent in the 13th century.
Use of turmeric in the Middle East is mainly for culinary purposes. Some dishes from the Middle East that use turmeric include the following:

- **Sfouf** – a Lebanese sweet cake made from semolina flour seasoned with turmeric powder
- **Khoresh** – Iranian stew dishes which extensively use turmeric as a flavoring
- **Chicken and Turmeric Rice** – Turmeric is used to make fragrant and colorful bright yellow rice, and this dish is widely popular in Middle Eastern countries

Europe

As previously mentioned, Arabs brought turmeric plants to Europe during the 13ᵗʰ century.
In 1280 AD, Marco Polo recorded that he has found a root plant resembling all the qualities of saffron. He noted that the herb can be used to dye cloth. This was the first known evidence that turmeric has reached Europe's Western civilization.

Europe's Doubt in Turmeric's Health Benefits

Turmeric was disregarded by Early Europeans in terms of medicinal use. They utilized turmeric just to dye fabrics, color medicines, and create turmeric paper used for testing a solution's acidity or alkalinity. They did not recognize turmeric use in health and well-being until the late 20ᵗʰ century.

Early 20ᵗʰ century Western herbalist Maude Grieve published a book called *A Modern Herbal* which briefly touched on turmeric's medicinal properties. She said that turmeric is simply a mild stimulant that was once used to treat jaundice and to test alkaloids and boric acid. She added that turmeric is rarely used in Western medicine and is simply used as a fabric coloring.

The earliest known recognition of turmeric as a medicinal herb came in the mid-20th century with the publication of Dr. Rudolph Weiss's book *Herbal Medicine* in 1961. Here, Dr. Weiss pointed out the efficacy of turmeric as a digestive system soother and liver problem remedy. However, he stressed that turmeric's yellowish pigment may cause irritation to the digestive tract linings, and thus cautioned the public about its use as a medicine.

The 1990s saw an increasing number of Western herbalists who promoted the use of turmeric as a medicinal plant. Herbalists such as Clark, Duke, Pederson, Murray, Hobbs, and Michael Castleman began introducing turmeric for the treatment of various illnesses of the liver and digestive tract, as well as for managing menstrual problems.

Modern Times

Nowadays, turmeric is produced in several countries such as Indonesia, China, the Philippines, Haiti, Jamaica, Nigeria, Costa Rica, Hawaii, and Kenya. India remains the top global produTurmeric is widely used in herbal medicine, with several food supplements and teas sprouting around and claiming to enhance health and well-being. Turmeric is still used in many cuisines across the globe today; it is a prized condiment that lends flavor and color to many dishes.

Chapter 3: The Amazing Benefits of Turmeric

Turmeric has been recently recognized as a "miracle spice" thanks to the many positive effects people have observed when taking this herbal root. Indeed, what the Indians and the Chinese have known since the earliest days proves to be true – turmeric has medicinal properties that help keep people healthy. This fact is now becoming clearer than ever, thanks to those who attest to turmeric's capacity to change their health.

Without further ado, here are some of turmeric's amazing positive benefits on human health and well-being:

Turmeric fights chronic inflammation

Turmeric has proven to be an effective anti-inflammatory that can alleviate inflammatory responses caused by chronic illnesses. Curcumin, the compound that gives turmeric its bright yellow color, is said to be responsible for this anti-inflammatory action.

A study conducted in 2009 found out that turmeric effectively reduces inflammation. The inflammation was caused by several diseases such as arthritis, inflammatory bowel disease, chronic anterior uveitis, pancreatitis, and certain cancer types. Arthritis patients respond especially well to turmeric and curcumin.

NF-kB is a molecule that goes deep into the cells' nuclei and activates genes related to inflammation. Turmeric's curcumin content binds to these molecules and prevents them from reaching the nuclei, hence stopping the inflammation response before it is actually triggered.

Another good thing about turmeric is that it fights inflammation without the usual side effects of corticosteroids, NSAIDs, and other types of anti-inflammatory medication.

Turmeric helps prevent abnormal blood clot formation

Formation of blood clots within the body's blood vessels is a natural and important part of the inflammation process. For instance, when you accidentally cut your finger, blood rushes out uncontrollably from the cut site. But after a few seconds, a blood component called *platelets* come together at the site of the cut and form a clot to help stop the bleeding.

This mechanism is known as *platelet aggregation*.

However, blood clot formation can be a cause of concern when abnormal amounts of clots form, get dislodged, travel through the veins and arteries, and can potentially impede blood flow to a certain body part if they get stuck in one vessel. Clots can also clump together to form huge ones that could be dangerous to your health.

Turmeric steps in to prevent excessive blood clot formation by interfering with platelet aggregation. Curcumin content in turmeric stops the platelet's action of concentrating in one area to form a new blood clot, hence greatly reducing the risk of abnormal blood clot formation. Curcumin does this by affecting the synthesis of *thromboxane*, a molecule included in the inflammatory process that stimulates blood clot formation.

Turmeric is recommended for people with viscous blood which predisposes them to frequent blood clots, such as diabetic persons. People with thinned blood should avoid using turmeric, as this may worsen their symptoms and put them at risk for severe bleeding.

Turmeric protects cells from damage & halts premature aging

Premature aging happens when the body experiences oxidative damage. Turmeric interferes with oxidative damage by building up a significantly strong army of antioxidants to fight off free radicals causing the damage.

Free radicals are molecules that react with organic substances such as DNA, proteins, and fatty acids. The chemical reaction between these free radicals and the body's organic substances creates oxidative damage. The result is dulled body tissues which make them prone to accelerated aging.

Widespread cellular damage can be stopped if the free radicals can be neutralized so that they don't interact with organic body substances. Turmeric's molecular structure allows it to neutralize free radicals, hence protecting cells from premature aging caused by oxidative damage and detoxifying the body as well. Studies also show that turmeric appears to stimulate the body to produce its own antioxidants. So not only does turmeric fight off free radicals, it also increases the antioxidants in the body to help fight off oxidative damage.

Turmeric protects the brain from damage and illnesses

Turmeric can increase the levels of *Brain-Derived Neurotropic Factor (BDNF)* in the brain. BDNF is an important substance that helps neurons communicate effectively with each other. Having low levels of BDNF in the brain is linked to various brain illnesses, such as Alzheimer's disease and depression.

Several animal trials have seen turmeric's potential to become a brain protectant. In these studies, animals that were given turmeric had significantly reduced symptoms of depression and had boosted brain function levels.

Studies also showed that curcumin found in turmeric improved the development of new brain cells in rats. This leads to better cognition and protection from degenerative brain illnesses like Alzheimer's disease.

Turmeric is indeed promising for brain health. However, more human trials should be done to finally prove this interesting health benefit.

Turmeric can control various types of pain

Studies in both humans and animals have shown the efficacy of turmeric as a natural pain reliever. Turmeric's effects on the following types of pain have been studied and were all rather promising:

- Sciatic nerve pain

- Arthritis pain

- Neuropathic pain

- Post-operative pain

- Pain from burns

- Pain arising from dental issues

- Pain associated with wounds

- Diabetic pain

Turmeric's effects on the brain also helps in diminishing anxiety and depression related to pain.

Turmeric may help diminish cancer

Turmeric has potential in alleviating and preventing cancer. Several studies have been carried out, showing the positive effects of turmeric use against cancer cells.

A 2013 clinical trial included turmeric and curcumin use to the conventional chemotherapy treatments that cancer patients use. Researchers then concluded that a combined therapy could be more powerful than standalone chemotherapy.

Several laboratory studies seem to verify the 2013 independent study on combined turmeric and chemotherapy use, emphasizing the role of turmeric in killing cancer cells.

Laboratory studies pitted turmeric-derived curcumin against cancer cells and found out that the cancer cells have died and stopped proliferating.

Specific types of cancer cell groups are shown to respond positively to turmeric:

- Stomach cancer

- Skin cancer

- Breast cancer

- Bowel cancer

Here are the mechanisms by which turmeric-derived curcumin appears to work in stopping cancer cell growth:

- Turmeric can stimulate a gene that inhibits growth of tumors.

- Turmeric cuts off blood supply to cancer cells through the inhibition of vascular epithelial cells. This leads to cancer cell death and prevention of cancer stem cell regrowth.

- Migration of cancer cells from one organ to another *(metastasis)* is halted by turmeric and its curcumin content.

- Inflammation enzyme *COX-2* can lead to cancer, and turmeric can help inhibit its action.

While all these information about turmeric's positive effects seem largely promising, more scientific studies are needed to completely validate turmeric's effects on cancer.

Turmeric helps in weight loss and stops obesity

The anti-inflammatory properties of turmeric can also help combat obesity and aid in weight loss. A study has revealed that turmeric's curcumin can help slow down the growth of fat cells in the body through its anti-inflammatory action.

Obesity may actually be viewed as a long-term metabolic inflammation. Turmeric's inhibition of the *NF-kB* substance helps reduce fat proliferation in the cells and lowers obesity's inflammation response in the body.

Turmeric also helps the liver in detoxifying the body. It aids in getting rid of *xenobiotics*, toxins arising from the environment and the diet. As the body is cleansed of these toxins, there's a greater chance for weight loss to occur.

Chapter 4: Turmeric & Curcumin

You may often hear the words turmeric and curcumin being used together. And if you may notice, curcumin often appeared in the previous chapters almost as much as turmeric does. But what really is turmeric and curcumin, how do they relate to each other, and what are their differences?

Turmeric and Curcumin Defined and Differentiated

Is turmeric and curcumin the same? This question perpetually lingers in the minds of curious people who want to learn more about turmeric's health benefits.
Strictly speaking, turmeric and curcumin are not the same. Here's why:

- Turmeric is the rhizomatic root of the *Curcuma longa* plant. It's that cylindrical brown root with a bright yellow-orange flesh. Turmeric can also refer to the powdered form which is used as a spice and condiment in the culinary world.

- On the other hand, curcumin is a substance that is found within turmeric. Curcumin is that compound which gives turmeric its distinct bright color.

Curcumin is also the active compound that gives turmeric most of its health properties. A typical turmeric root contains around 2-5% of curcumin.

In simple terms, turmeric is a source of curcumin. You can extract curcumin compounds from turmeric roots. In that sense, the two are distinct from one another. Turmeric is the actual root or powder, while curcumin is the naturally-occurring compound contained within turmeric.

Curcumin was actually identified as a separate substance in the year 1815 and its chemical structure was successfully mapped in 1910. But why is turmeric often mistaken to be the same as curcumin? The two terms are often interchangeably used because they are so closely related together in the sense that curcumin is actually inside turmeric.

Delving Deeper into Curcumin

You now know the difference between turmeric and curcumin. So, it's time to learn more about curcumin.

Turmeric (both in fresh and powdered forms) naturally contains a family of chemicals collectively known as *curcuminoids*. This chemical family is composed of polyphenolic phytochemical substances that give off a bright yellow hue. Curcuminoids present in turmeric include the following:

- Cyclocurcumin

- Desmethoxycurcumin

- Bisdemethoxycurcumin

- Curcumin

Among these four, the most abundant in Turmeric is Curcumin. It makes up around 77% of turmeric's chemical composition. Desmethoxycurcumin comes in second at 17%, followed by Bisdemethoxycurcumin and Cyclocurcumin at 3% each.

Curcumin is chemically known as a *diarylheptanoid*. It is a fat-soluble compound with somewhat poor oral bioavailability, which means only a small amount of curcumin you ingest gets absorbed by the body. It also has a limited bioactivity, meaning it is chemically unstable and can be quickly metabolized by the body once ingested.

Despite these downsides, curcumin has been extensively tested to help treat conditions such as inflammation, heart problems, digestive concerns, pain, brain conditions, and cancer. No conclusive evidence to prove curcumin's effectiveness as a medical drug has been reached yet, but there are significant positive health changes seen in most of the studies undertaken.

Curcumin is widely recognized in alternative medicine. It is believed that curcumin can be taken with the following supplements to increase protection against certain conditions:

- *Garcinia indica (Garcinol)* – to help prevent most cancer types
- *DHA and fish oil* – to help prevent breast cancer
- *Soy isoflavones and Genistein* – to help prevent prostate cancer
- *Black pepper extracts* – to increase absorption and bioavailability

You can get your daily fix of curcumin from fresh turmeric roots and other processed turmeric products like powders and teas. However, be reminded that only 2-5% of curcumin is present in each average-sized turmeric root, and that your body absorbs even less amounts in the end. You might need a steady supply of fresh turmeric roots and include them in your daily meals in order to get health benefits from curcumin in the most natural way.

Curcumin is commercially available in powders, supplements, teas, and topical skincare products. It is generally safe to use – 8 grams per day for 3 to 4 months is the safest and most common dosage for curcumin. Larger doses may cause the following adverse effects:

- Stomach cramps

- Diarrhea

- Mild nausea and vomiting

- Skin allergies (when used topically)

Pregnant and lactating women are advised to steer clear from curcumin use, as effects on the unborn child have not yet been extensively studied. Children are advised not to take turmeric continuously. Parents should seek the opinion of their healthcare provider before starting to give turmeric to their kids on a regular basis.

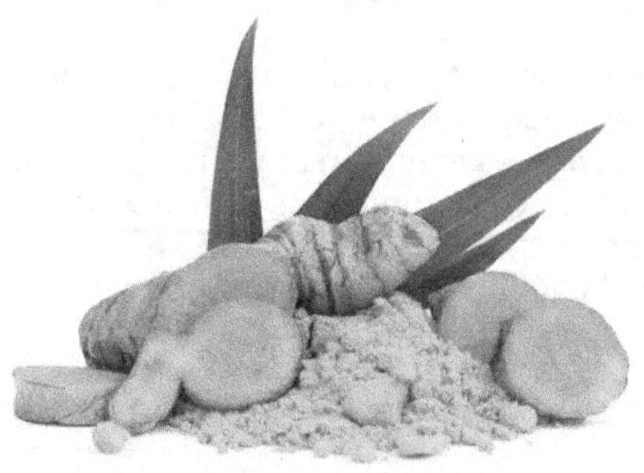

Chapter 5:   How to Cook with Turmeric Correctly

Now that you know how beneficial turmeric can be for your health, it's time to buff up your turmeric intake naturally by including this tasty root in your daily dishes. But you just don't include turmeric in everything you cook! Learn how to cook with turmeric correctly using this simple guide.

Increasing Turmeric and Curcumin Absorption

As previously said, not all the curcumin that comes from eating turmeric gets absorbed by the body. Only a fraction of this healthy compound gets into your blood and tissues.
But there are some ways to raise the absorption level of turmeric in the body:

- **Add a pinch of black pepper extracts.**

  - Black pepper extracts contain an active component called *piperine*. It's the compound responsible for black pepper's pungent flavor and aroma. Black pepper contains around 5% of piperine.

- Piperine increases curcumin absorption in the bloodstream by inhibiting the liver's active ability to metabolize curcumin quickly. Piperine can raise the amount of curcumin in the body by up to 2000%.
- It is recommended to take around ¼ teaspoon of black pepper extract together with a teaspoon of turmeric powder to enhance absorption. That's just about a pinch of black pepper extract.
- Here's something interesting – curry uses lots of turmeric powder and black pepper. That means you get lots of curcumin absorbed in your body when you eat curries! Not only does the dish taste even more delicious, it becomes genuinely healthy as well.

- **Infuse your turmeric dishes with some oils and fat.**

  o Curcumin is fat soluble. Hence, when you add a bit of fat or oil on your turmeric dishes, you increase the chances of curcumin getting dissolved in fat, making it easier for the compound to get retained in your digestive system and eventually be absorbed in your body.

- o Just a few drops of vegetable oil or butter in your dishes will tremendously help improve curcumin absorption. You don't have to go all out and drench your dishes in fat; as always, moderation is key.

- **Eat fresh turmeric.**

  - o Consuming fresh turmeric roots ups the chances of absorption as compared to using powder in your dishes. It's because natural oils are released as fresh turmeric is being eaten. Again, oil dissolves the curcumin and makes it easier for the digestive tract to absorb. The liver won't readily metabolize curcumin wrapped in its natural oils.

  - o Chop up your turmeric roots and toss them into vegetable salads. Munch on them as much as you like. It's one of the best ways to ramp up your curcumin intake.

It's worth mentioning that in India, they slather fresh turmeric with fat and peppercorns, then eat it raw or use them in curry dishes. Rarely do they use ground turmeric powders. If they do, they make sure to use homemade ground turmeric powders. Maybe this is a coincidence, but isn't it good to think that using a bit of fat and a pinch of pepper on turmeric dishes not only makes them appetizing, but it makes them healthier, too?

Turning Turmeric into Powder

Sometimes, you'll need to quickly pop in some turmeric powder as you cook. Or maybe your recipe calls for ground turmeric instead of fresh chunks or grated turmeric. Or perhaps you've grown too much turmeric in your backyard and need to turn some of them into powder for more practical uses and for a longer shelf life.

In any case, you can have your fresh turmeric roots turned into homemade powder by following these simple steps:

1. Wash your freshly-harvested turmeric rhizomes thoroughly. Take out excess soil, long roots, and leaves. Wash them until all you see left are the bulbs and fingers of the turmeric.
2. Place them on a pan and cover with large leaves. Set aside for one entire day. This step is part of a traditional method of drying; you may skip this step if you're running out of time.
3. Boil the turmeric rhizomes in a large pot for 45 minutes, according to the recommendations of The Indian Institute of Spice Research and the Agricultural Research Center. As you boil, you'll smell the aroma and notice some froth.

4. Check for softness before taking the rhizomes out of the heat. Gently pierce the rhizomes using a small piece of wooden cooking utensil. Assess the softness; the root should come off and break gently. It is crucial that the rhizomes are boiled to a proper softness or else they will become brittle.
5. Transfer to a clean pan and cut into small vertical pieces.
6. Lay them side by side on a flat surface and let them dry under sunlight. If there is no sunlight, you may also use your microwave oven to dry the rhizomes. Work batch by batch when using the microwave so that the rhizomes are completely dried.
7. After thorough drying, use a grinder to grind your turmeric rhizomes. Pass through a strainer, catch large particles, then grind again till every rhizome becomes powdery.
8. Transfer to an airtight jar and seal accordingly.

Your ground turmeric is now ready to be used.

Not Just for Curries

Turmeric can be used for a variety of delicious dishes. You can cook and add turmeric (fresh or ground – it's up to you) to the following dishes:

- Stews

- Soups

- Cooked rice

- Stir-fried vegetables

- Pancakes

- Egg dishes, frittatas, quiche

- Pumpkin pies

- Marinades for chicken, beef, and fish recipes

- Smoothies

- Fresh pressed juices

There are no limitations to where you can use turmeric for cooking.

Chapter 6: Turmeric Recipes

Excited to cook with turmeric? Get started with some of these simple recipes. Feel free to adjust the ingredients to suit how many servings you would like to prepare.

Turmeric Omelet

This is an easy-to-prepare breakfast that you can whip up in under 15 minutes. Yields two servings.

Ingredients:

- 4 large eggs
- 1/8 teaspoon turmeric powder
- 3/8 teaspoon sea salt/kosher salt
- 2 green onions, finely chopped
- ¼ cup medium-sized tomato, diced
- ¼ cup brown mustard seeds
- 1 tablespoon olive oil
- Black pepper to taste

Procedure:

1. Break eggs in a bowl and whisk together with salt.

2. Heat olive oil in a medium-sized skillet over medium heat. Place turmeric powder and mustard seeds. Cook for 30 seconds, continuously stirring until you hear and see the mustard seeds pop.
3. Add onions and cook until softened.
4. Add tomatoes and cook for a minute or until soft.
5. Pour whisked eggs into the pan and cook for about two minutes or until edges begin to set. Ensure that the eggs are set evenly as it cooks.
6. Lift the egg to the other side and cook for another two minutes.
7. Use a spatula to loosen the omelet from the pan and fold it into half.
8. Slide the folded omelet onto a plate, cut into half, and top with black pepper.

Stir-Fry Vegetables with Turmeric

This Indian-inspired stir-fry dish uses cabbage and turmeric as the star ingredients. It's a tasty, succulent, and extremely healthy vegetarian dish perfect for lunch and dinner. Yields 6 servings (around 1 1/3 cups each).

Ingredients:

- 1 head of a 3 ½ pound green cabbage, cored and chopped finely
- 3 red peppers, seeded and chopped finely
- 3 orange peppers, seeded and chopped finely
- 3 dried red chilies
- 1 teaspoon ground turmeric & 1 teaspoon black mustard seeds
- 24 pieces curry leaves (fresh or frozen will both do)
- 1 cup green peas
- 1 cup cilantro, chopped coarsely
- 3 tablespoons canola oil
- 1 ½ teaspoon cumin seeds
- 1 tablespoon flaked unsweetened coconut
- ¾ teaspoon sea salt/kosher salt
- Black pepper to taste

Procedure:
1. Heat canola oil in a skillet over medium high heat.
2. Combine together coconut, cumin, turmeric powder, mustard seeds, curry leaves, and chilies. Cook for 3 minutes with occasional stirring. Let chilies turn brown.
3. Add bell peppers, peas, and cabbage. Sauté for 5 minutes until the cabbage turns tender but still crisp.
4. Add in cilantro, salt, and a pinch of black pepper. Stir well.
5. Serve hot in small bowls.

Kielbasa Rice with Chicken

Brightly colored rice from the turmeric comes together with chicken broth, sausage, and turkey kielbasa. Not only is this dish a feast for the eyes, it's definitely a treat for your taste buds as well. Yields 3 to 4 servings.

Ingredients:

- 2 cups long grain parboiled rice
- 8 ounces chicken thighs (skinless and boneless), cut into small bite-sized pieces
- 2 cups chicken broth
- 8 ounces turkey kielbasa, cut into half-inch pieces
- 1/8 teaspoon ground turmeric
- 1 cup onion, chopped finely and 1 cup green bell pepper, chopped finely
- ½ cup green peas
- 1 tablespoon garlic, minced
- ¼ cup stuffed manzanilla or green olives, sliced and pitted
- 2 teaspoons olive oil with Kosher salt and black pepper to taste

Procedure:
1. Heat a saucepan over medium heat. Combine the broth, kielbasa, and turmeric. Let the mixture boil.

2. Stir in rice, cover, then reduce heat to low.
    Let simmer for 5 minutes, then remove
    from heat and set aside.

3. Heat olive oil in another large skillet over
    high heat.

4. Add chicken bits and cook for 2 minutes
    until brownish in color.

5. Add in onions and bell pepper. Sauté until
    tender.

6. Add peas, garlic, and olives. Sauté for a
    minute.

7. Add in the rice, broth, and kielbasa
    mixture. Mix thoroughly and cook for a
    minute until rice is thoroughly heated.

8. Season with a pinch of sea salt and black
    pepper. Serve hot on bowls.

Curry with Veggies, Turmeric & Coconut Milk

A curry recipe would definitely make it to this book! Turmeric and coconut lend an earthy yet rich flavor to this delicious curry recipe. Throw in some vegetables, and you have a healthy course for dinner tonight. Yields 4 servings.
Ingredients:

- 1 medium-sized eggplant, diced
- 1 carrot, diced
- 1 red bell pepper, diced
- 1 yellow bell pepper, diced
- 1 zucchini, diced
- 1 clove garlic, chopped finely
- 1 white onion, chopped finely
- 2 teaspoons ground turmeric
- ½ teaspoon ground coriander
- ½ teaspoon curry powder
- ½ can chickpeas, drained and rinsed
- 1 can coconut milk
- 2 tablespoons golden sultanas
- 2 teaspoons olive oil
- Salt and black pepper to taste
- Chopped fresh coriander for garnish

Procedure:
1. Heat olive oil on a large pot over medium high heat.

2. Sauté onions until soft. Add garlic, carrots, and eggplant. Cook for 5 minutes.

3. Add the rest of the vegetables, as well as turmeric, curry powder, and coriander. Mix and cook for 2 to 3 minutes.

4. Stir in coconut milk. Reduce heat, and cover pot. Simmer for 20 minutes.

5. Around 5 minutes before cooking time ends, pop in the sultanas.

6. Season with some salt and pepper. Serve on bowls and top with fresh coriander to garnish.

Turmeric Flavored Chicken Soup

Ingredients:

- 1.5kg organic chicken
- 1 small head garlic, sliced horizontally, plus 3 garlic cloves, finely chopped, extra
- 2 tea spoon turmeric
- 5cm-piece ginger, peeled, chopped, plus 1 table spoon finely chopped, extra
- 1 long fresh red chilli, finely chopped
- 270ml can coconut milk
- 200g packet fresh sweet potato noodles (you might have to make this yourself)
- 1 tsp white peppercorns
- 1 tbsp coconut oil or olive oil
- 1-2 tbsp tamari, to taste
- 1 lime, juiced, plus wedges, extra, to serve
- Fresh coriander sprigs, to serve

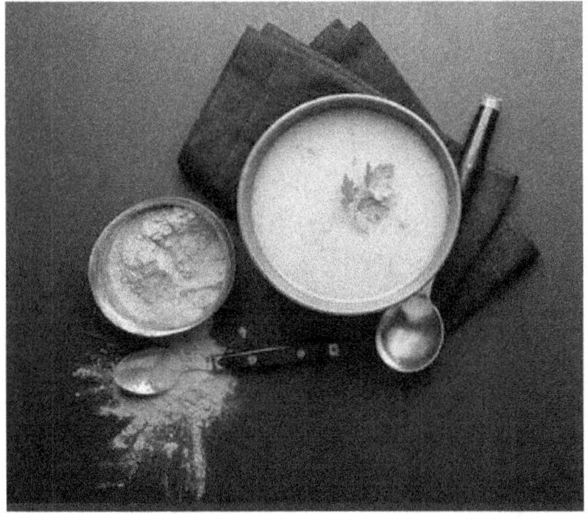

Procedure:

1. Place the chicken in a stockpot. Add 4L (16 cups) water to cover. Bring to the boil, over high heat, skimming and discarding any fat that comes to the surface. Reduce heat to low.
2. Add the garlic, ginger, and peppercorns. Simmer, skimming occasionally, for 1½ hours or until the chicken is very tender. Transfer chicken to a plate and set aside to cool. Coarsely shred the meat and discard the skin and bones. Strain the chicken stock, discarding the solids and reserving the liquid.
3. Heat the coconut oil in a large saucepan.
4. Add the chili, extra garlic and extra ginger. Cook, stirring, for 2 minutes or until aromatic.
5. Stir in the turmeric. Cook, stirring, for 1 minute or until aromatic. Slowly pour in the reserved chicken stock. Add the coconut milk. Simmer for 20 minutes or until reduced slightly.
6. Add the sweet potato noodles and shredded chicken and simmer for 5 minutes or until zoodles are tender. Stir in the tamari and lime juice. Season to taste. Divide among serving bowls. Top with coriander and serve with extra lime wedges.

Middle Eastern Turmeric Chicken with Rice

Ingredients:
For the Chicken

- 5 skin on, bone in, chicken thighs
- 2 tablespoons of lemon juice
- 2 table spoons of turmeric powder
- 1 table spoon of cumin
- ½ table spoon of curry
- 1 tbsp dried oregano
- 4 garlic cloves, minced
- 1 tea spoon of salt
- 1 tea spoon of black pepper

For the Rice

- 2 tbsp olive oil, divided
- 1 small onion, finely chopped
- 1 clove of garlic, finely minced
- 1½ cups basmati rice
- 1½ cups chicken broth
- 1 cup water
- 1 tbsp dried oregano
- 1 tbsp of turmeric powder
- 1 teaspoon salt
- 1 tea spoon of cumin

Procedure:

1. Combine the chicken and all the ingredients for the chicken in a large resealable bag, and let it marinade for at least 30 minutes (preferably over night for more flavor).
2. Preheat the oven to 220°C.
3. In a large oven safe skillet, heat 1 tbsp of olive oil over medium high heat. Place the chicken in the skillet skin side down and cook until golden brown (about 3-5 minutes), then flip over and cook the other side until golden brown (another 3-5 minutes).
4. Remove the chicken and set aside.
5. Remove any black or burnt bits from the pan and add another tablespoon of olive oil to the pan over medium high heat.
6. Add the onions to the skillet with the oregano, turmeric, and cumin. Sauté until the onions become translucent.
7. Add the garlic and basmati rice and sauté for 1 minute, just until the rice begins to turn golden.
8. Add the chicken broth, water, and salt and bring to a simmer. Place the cooked chicken thighs directly on top of the rice and liquid. Once the liquid has begun to simmer, cover with a lid, and transfer to the oven to continue cooking.

9. Bake in the oven for 30 minutes. After 30
   minutes, remove the lid and continue to
   bake for an additional 15 minutes, until all
   the liquid has been absorbed.
10. Remove from the oven and let sit for 10
   minutes before serving. Garnish with grilled
   lemon slice, and fresh parsley.

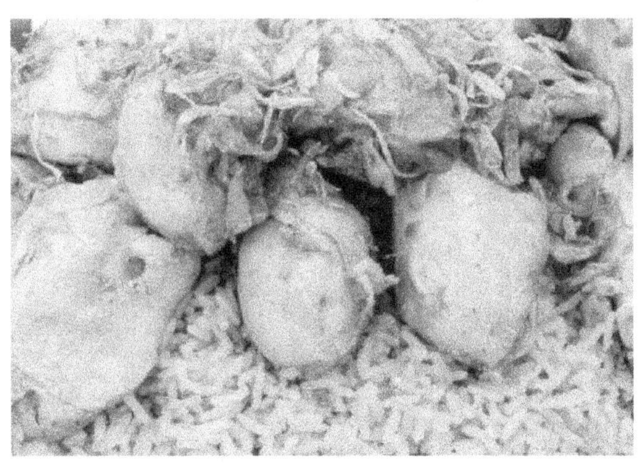

Turmeric Chicken Pizza with a Chickpea Flatbread Base

This recipe makes 4 mini pizzas.

Ingredients:

For Chicken Marinade

- ¼ cup honey
  3 tablespoons whole grain mustard
- 2 tablespoons of smooth Dijon mustard
- 2 tablespoons of olive oil
- 1 tablespoon of turmeric
- 1 tablespoon of minced garlic
- Salt to season
- 2 chicken breasts, sliced

For Base

- 2 cups chickpea flour
- 1 cup water
- 1 tablespoon of olive oil
- A Pinch of salt

Procedure:

For the Base

1. Preheat oven to 180°C.
2. Line a baking tray with baking paper.

3. In a medium bowl, stir together the chickpea flour, water, olive oil and salt until well mixed.
4. Spread mixture out into rounds (depending on size of base desired).
5. Bake for 5–10 minutes or until crust is slightly crispy.
6. Remove from the oven, turn over and peel paper away from the base.

For the Chicken Marinade

1. In a small bowl, whisk together all the marinade ingredients (honey through salt).
2. Pour marinade into a large zip lock bag and ass chicken to the bag and shake to ensure all the chicken is coated in the marinade. If time allows, place bag of chicken in the refrigerator to marinate for at least 2 hours.
3. Heat a non-stick pan, or outdoor grill over medium heat with about a teaspoon of oil and cook/grill chicken on each side until golden, crispy, and cooked through.

Cover bases with your favorite toppings and bake for another 2-3 minutes or until cheese has melted.

Chapter 7: Turmeric Beverages & Sweets

Mango, Ginger & Turmeric Smoothie

Ingredients:

- 2in piece of Ginger
- 3/4 cup Mango (fresh or frozen)
- 1 Banana
- 1/4 cup Oats
- 1 teaspoon Honey
- 1 teaspoon Turmeric
- 1/4 cup Greek Yogurt
- 3/4 cup Milk of your choice (cows, soy, almond, rice, etc.)

Procedure:

Just like all other smoothies. Put all of the ingredients together in a blender.

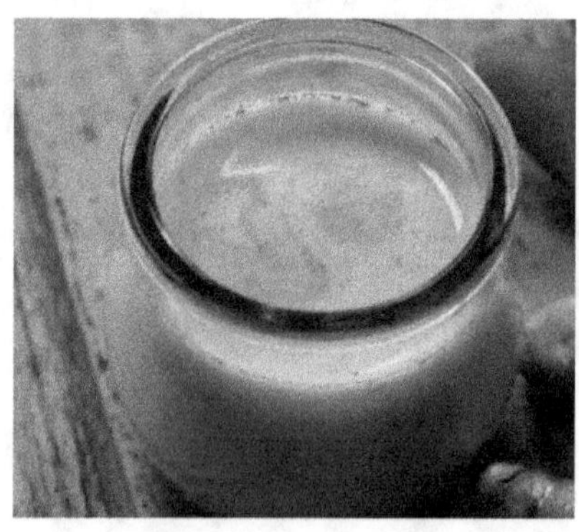

Turmeric Summer Fruit Smoothie

Ingredients:

- 1 tablespoon coconut oil
- 1 cup hemp or coconut milk
- ½ cup frozen pineapple
- ½ teaspoon turmeric (or 1 tsp. turmeric)
- 1 fresh banana
- ½ teaspoon ginger
- ½ teaspoon cinnamon
- 1 teaspoon chia seeds

Procedure:

Just like all other smoothies. Put all of the ingredients together in a blender. Mix until you get that sweet homogenous mixture.

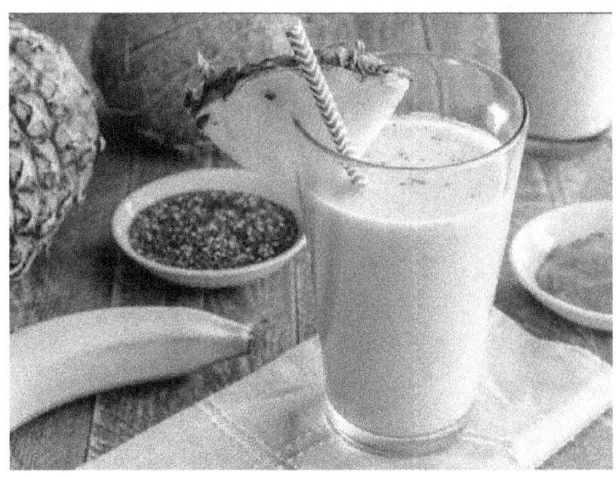

Turmeric Golden Milk

You will first need to make up some Turmeric Paste before making your Golden Milk.

Turmeric Paste Recipe

Ingredients:

- 1/2 Cup of organic turmeric powder
- 1/2 Teaspoon ground black pepper
- 1 Cup filtered water
- 1/3 Cup raw coconut oil

Procedure:

1. Place turmeric and water in a pan, stirring over a gentle heat until you have a thick paste. This should take about 7-10 minutes and you may need to add additional water along the way.
2. Add the freshly ground pepper and oil AT THE END of cooking. Stir well (a whisk is ideal) to incorporate the oil and allow to cool.

Golden Milk Recipe

Ingredients:

- 1 Cup milk
  (almond, coconut, or organic cow's milk)
- 1 Teaspoon raw organic coconut oil
- ¼ Teaspoon turmeric paste
  (more can be added for personal taste preference)
- Sweeten with honey
  (to taste)

Procedure:

1. Combine all ingredients except honey in a small saucepan.
2. Cook on medium heat, stirring constantly.
3. When completely blended and hot (but not boiling) remove from heat and add honey to taste, stirring until dissolved.

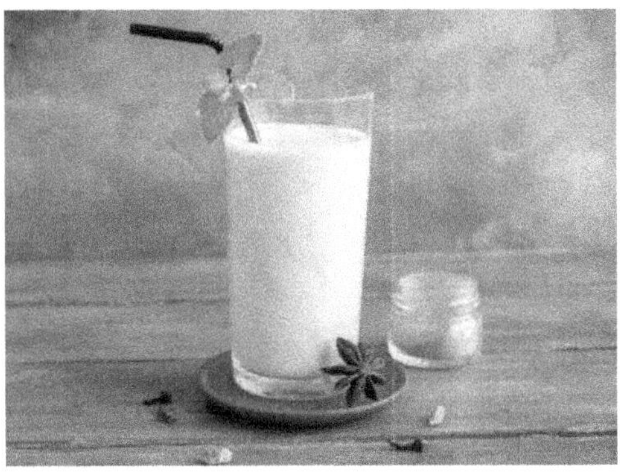

Turmeric Ginger Tea

Ingredients:

This is a simple sweet and milky tea with
warming spices. You can use regular milk, or
the nut milk of your choice.

- 1 cup water
- 1/4 teaspoon ground turmeric
- 1/4 teaspoon ground ginger
- 1/8 teaspoon ground cardamom
- 2 tablespoons milk
- Maple syrup to taste

Procedure:

Bring water to boil with turmeric and ginger,
turn down heat and simmer for 5 minutes.
Stir in milk and maple to taste, serve.

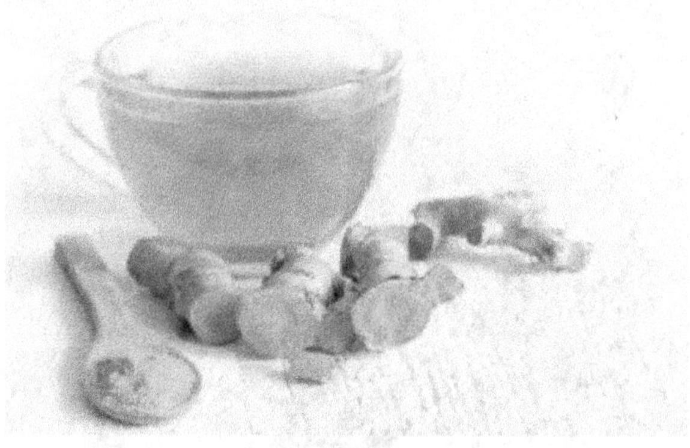

Turmeric Super Booster

Ingredients:

- 2 tablespoon turmeric powder
- 6 tablespoons raw unfiltered apple cider vinegar
- 3 – 4 tablespoons local raw honey
- 1 lemon, juice and zest
- ½ teaspoon black pepper

Procedure:

1. Whisk your turmeric in a small mixing bowl or grind lightly with a mortar and pestle to loosen clumps, and smooth into a fine powder.
2. Next add in the apple cider vinegar, honey, lemon juice and zest and pepper. Stir until smooth.
3. Consume as a warm tonic, by mixing 1 tablespoon with a large mug of warm water. Or on top of toast or as a baked good topping. Add a tablespoon or two into your green juice or blend it into your smoothie.

Turmeric and Lime Tonic

Ingredients:

- 3 Cups coconut water
- ½ inch Fresh grated ginger (you can add more to your personal preference of taste)
- 1 Lime cut in quarters and squeezed
- 1 Tablespoon turmeric powder
- 1/4 Teaspoon cardamom
- 2 Teaspoons honey
- Cayenne pepper to taste

Procedure:

Combine ingredients in a sealable container, shake well and refrigerate overnight.
Shake well before serving.

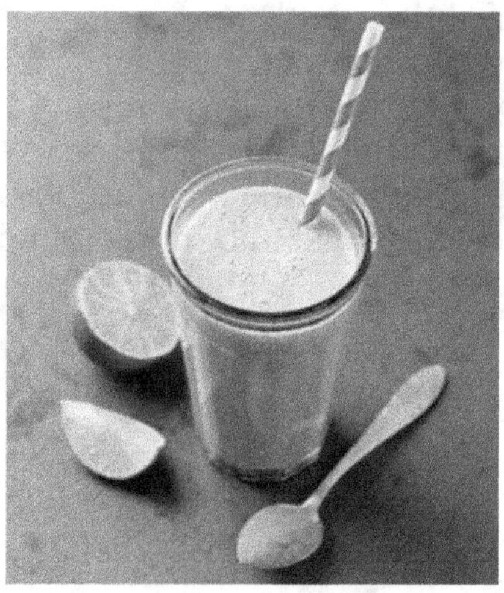

Turmeric Ice Cream

Please note this recipe serves 8.

Ingredients:

- 2 x cans of full fat coconut milk or coconut cream
- 4 quarter-size slices fresh ginger
- 1/4 cup maple syrup
- Pinch sea salt
- 2 tsp ground turmeric
- 1/2 teaspoon ground cinnamon
- 1/8th teaspoon black pepper
- 1 tsp pure vanilla extract
- *optional:* 1/8th teaspoon cardamom
- *optional:* 2 Tablespoons of (30 ml) olive oil
- *optional:* 1/4 cup chopped candied ginger

Procedure:

1. The day or night before, place your ice cream churning bowl in the freezer to properly chill (see notes if you don't have an ice cream maker). Also, add coconut milk, fresh ginger, maple syrup, sea salt, turmeric, cinnamon, pepper, and cardamom (optional) to a large saucepan and heat over medium heat.

2. Bring to a simmer (not a boil), whisking
    thoroughly to combine ingredients. Then,
    remove from heat and add vanilla extract.
    Whisk once more to combine.
3. Taste and adjust flavor as needed, adding
    in more turmeric for intense turmeric
    flavor, cinnamon for warmth, maple
    syrup for sweetness, or salt to balance the
    flavors.
4. Transfer mixture (including the whole
    ginger slices) to a mixing bowl and let
    cool to room temperature. Then cover
    and chill in refrigerator overnight, or for
    at least 4-6 hours.
5. The following day, use a spoon (or
    strainer) to remove the ginger. At this
    time, you can also add olive oil for extra
    creaminess by whisking in thoroughly to
    combine.
6. Add to ice cream maker and churn
    according to manufacturer's instructions
    – about 20-30 minutes. It should look
    like soft serve.
7. While it's churning, chop up your candied
    ginger (optional). In the last few minutes
    of churning, add in the ginger to
    incorporate.
8. Once churned, transfer the ice cream to a
    large freezer-safe container (such as a
    parchment-lined loaf pan) and use a
    spoon to smooth the top.

9. Cover securely and freeze for at least 4-6 hours or until firm. Set out for 10 minutes before serving to soften and use a hot ice cream scoop (warmed in hot water) to ease scooping.
10. Will keep in the freezer for up to 10 days or more, though best within the first 7 days. Enjoy this as a lighter dessert with some serious health benefits!

*Please note that if you don't have an ice cream maker, you can add the chilled mixture to a freezer safe container and place in the freezer. Remove from freezer every 1-2 hours and stir vigorously to incorporate air. This won't make it as light and airy as an ice cream maker, but it works in a pinch!

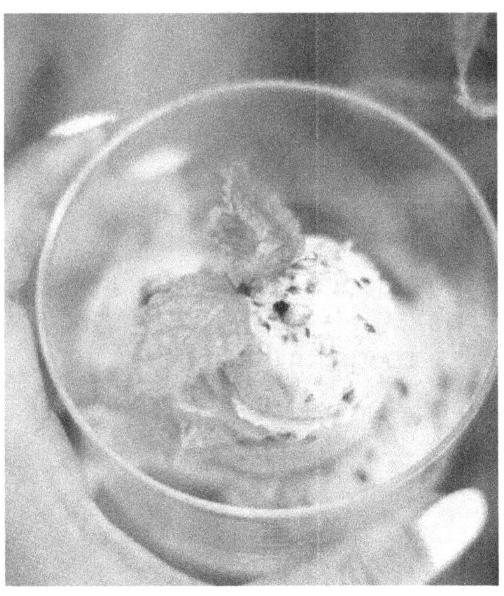

Turmeric & Mango Vegan Cheesecake

Ingredients:

Base

- 1¼ cups almonds
- ½ cup shredded coconut
- ¾ cup dates
- Zest of 1 lemon
- ½ teaspoon vanilla powder
- ¼ teaspoon sea salt
- 1 tablespoon coconut oil (melted)

Filling

- 2 ½ cups cashews (soaked 2 hours, drained, and rinsed)
- 1 cup coconut milk
- 1 cup coconut oil (melted)
- Juice and flesh of ½ lemon
- ¼ cup coconut nectar
- 1 tsp honey or maple syrup
- ¼ teaspoon sea salt
- 2 cups mango flesh (fresh if possible, chopped)
- 2 teaspoons turmeric

Procedure:

1. To make the base, blend almonds and shredded coconut in a food processor until well chopped but still with some chunky texture.
2. Add dates one by one while motor is still running. Then add remaining base ingredients and blend until well combined.
3. Pour the mixture into a 20cm spring form cake tin with the base of the tin lined with baking paper. Press the mixture down with a spatula until firm and flat. Place in the freezer to firm.
4. Blend all the filling ingredients, except mango and turmeric, in a food processor or blender until completely smooth, scraping down the inside of the food processor a few times to remove lumps. The mixture should be completely smooth like a thick cream.
5. Pour half of the cream mixture into a bowl and set aside. Then, add the mango and turmeric to the remaining cream mixture in the blender, and process until well combined.
6. Remove base from freezer and, using one quarter of the plain cream mixture, dollop generous spoonful's on top of the base.

7. Repeat this with dollops of one quarter of the mango mixture, then continue layering in this way until both mixtures have been used up.

8. Using a chopstick, swirl figure-eight patterns through the mixture to create a swirling effect between the two creams. Don't over-swirl or you will end up with a completely light orange cheesecake.

9. Place in the freezer overnight. An hour before you want to serve it, remove from the tin and place in the fridge. This helps to maintain its lovely firm texture, like an Italian semi-freddo.

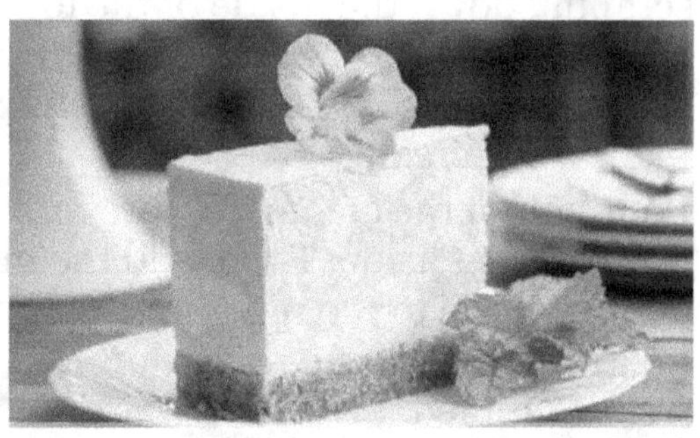

Delicious Golden Turmeric

Granola Clusters

Ingredients:

- 2 cups rolled oats, divided*
- ½ cup raw almonds
- ½ cup raw shelled sunflower seeds
- ¼ cup hemp seeds
- ½cup creamy unsalted almond butter
- ½ cup maple syrup
- ⅓ cup coconut oil
- 2 teaspoons pure vanilla extract
- 2 table spoons ground turmeric
- 1 teaspoon ground cinnamon
- ¼ teaspoon cardamom (optional)
- ¼ teaspoon fine grain sea salt

Procedure:

1. Preheat oven to 135 degrees C and line a large baking tray with baking paper.
2. Add ½ cup of the rolled oats and the almonds to a food processor and process for 1 minute or until the texture resembles a coarse flour.

Transfer to a large mixing bowl and add the remaining 1 ½ cups of rolled oats, sunflower seeds, and hemp seeds. Use a large wooden spoon to mix.

3. In a medium saucepan, whisk together the almond butter, maple syrup, coconut oil, vanilla, turmeric, cinnamon, cardamom (if using), and sea salt over low heat for 3 minutes or until smooth and glossy. Pour over the oat mixture and get stirring. Once every bit of the granola is evenly-coated, turn it out onto the lined baking tray and use the back of a spoon or spatula to spread it out into an even layer.

4. Bake for 15 minutes, rotate the pan back-to-front, and bake another 20 to 26 minutes. The granola is ready when it's wafting a toasted scent, the top is a very light golden-brown, and it feels firm but not yet crisp to the touch. Note: Granola doesn't become crisp and crunchy until it's had a chance to cool, so rely on look and scent more than touch or you'll end up with burnt granola. Once the granola is ready, remove the pan from the oven and place it on an oven-safe cooling rack to allow air to circulate beneath and around the pan to efficiently cool and crisp the granola.

5. Allow the granola to cool completely on the pan until it's not even the slightest bit warm to the touch.

If you start moving it around or try to break it into clusters while it's still warm, it will crumble. I recommend a minimum 45 minutes of cool time at room temperature but try to hold out for 1 hour if you can.

6. Once the granola is completely cool, break it into pieces of desired size and store in large airtight glass jars to maintain its crunch.
7. Serve over coconut yogurt with fresh berries, enjoy with generous splash of cold almond milk, or snack on the clusters straight from the jar.

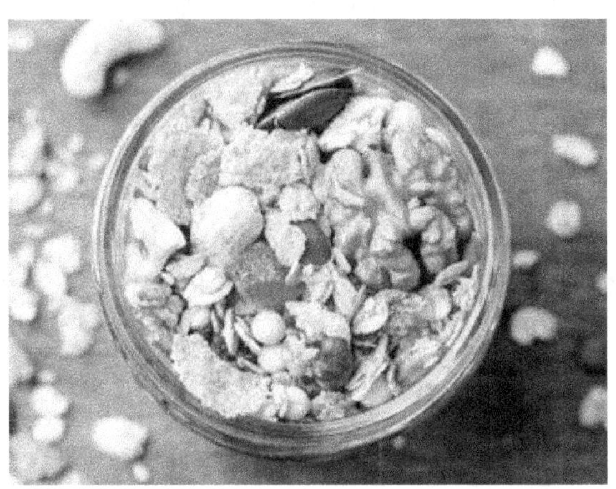

Conclusion

Thank you for reading my book on Turmeric, I hope the information I provided was able to help you understand more about the miracle spice and its great benefits for your health and well-being.

Please note however that when using turmeric, be careful of its color as it can easily stain hands, countertops and chopping boards. Therefore, you should immediately wash any area turmeric touches and consider wearing gloves to prevent staining your hands and fingers.

Well now, the next step is to go ahead and try some of the amazing recipes that I have included in this book and take some further action towards living a good healthy life. Turmeric is readily obtainable both in fresh and ground form; you can even grow it in your own garden! Utilize the power of this miracle spice in your kitchen and see your health gradually reach a higher level.

I wish you the best of luck!